Isometric Exercises for Pain Relief

Relieve Aches in Your Back, Neck, Knees and More Using Simple Static Contraction Exercises Without Equipment

Troy Vhodes

Copyright © 2024 by Troy Vhodes

Table of Contents

Introduction

In the realm of fitness, where sweat and determination converge, there exists a transformative approach to wellness that transcends traditional workouts. Imagine a journey where your body becomes a sculptor, crafting strength, resilience, and freedom from pain. Welcome to the world of isometric exercises – a realm where the simplicity of static contractions becomes a symphony of relief for aches that have lingered for too long.

Once upon a time, I found myself entangled in the web of discomfort and persistent pain. It was a struggle many of us know too well – the nagging ache in the back, the tension knotting up the neck, the soreness in the knees that seemingly refused to dissipate. Yet, amid this struggle, I stumbled upon a revelation that would change my fitness journey forever: isometric exercises for pain relief.

Let me share a personal anecdote that might resonate with you. Picture a time when every step felt like a burden, when the daily rituals were tainted by the shadow of pain. That was my reality until the day I discovered the incredible potential of isometric training. The simplicity of static contraction exercises became my sanctuary, a refuge where the pain slowly dissipated, and strength emerged as my newfound ally.

Embark with me on a journey that goes beyond the conventional fitness narrative. Imagine the scenes of your life where pain no longer holds sway –

a morning without stiffness, an afternoon without tension, and a night without the ghostly whispers of discomfort. This is the promise of isometric exercises for pain relief, a promise I extend to you with enthusiasm and conviction.

Did you know that isometric exercises are not just about physical transformation, but also a gateway to holistic well-being? It's a fact – backed by science and echoed by those who have embraced this unique fitness approach. As we delve into the world of isometrics, we unlock a path to not only sculpt our bodies but also nurture our mental and emotional resilience.

"What if you could bid farewell to aches and pains with just a few minutes of simple static contractions each day?" It's not a hypothetical question; it's an invitation to a reality that awaits you within these pages. As we explore the uniqueness of isometric exercises, you'll discover a training method that leverages the power of your bodyweight, eliminating the need for complex equipment or expensive gym memberships.

In the pages that follow, I offer you a sneak peek into the treasures that await: techniques that target specific pain points, tips to maximize your isometric practice, and carefully crafted programs that cater to various fitness levels. This guide is not just a collection of exercises; it's a roadmap to a pain-free, empowered existence.

Chapter 1
The Power of Isometric Training
Benefits of Isometric Exercises

Welcome to the first chapter of our journey into the transformative world of isometric training! Grab a seat, get comfortable, and let's dive into the magic that makes isometric exercises a game-changer in your quest for pain relief and strength.

Benefits of Isometric Exercises

Alright, let's cut to the chase - why should you care about isometric exercises? Well, it's not just about breaking a sweat (though you'll definitely do that). Imagine sculpting your body with the precision of a master craftsman, focusing on specific muscles to alleviate pain and boost strength.

Think of isometrics as your secret weapon against the aches that have been nagging you. Picture this: a world where your back no longer protests every time you bend down, where your neck and shoulders feel light as a feather, and where your knees cease their creaking protest. Isometrics isn't just a workout; it's a remedy, a solution, and a ticket to a more comfortable, pain-free existence.

How Isometrics Differ from Other Exercise Forms & Scientific Basis for Pain Relief through Isometrics

Now, you might be wondering, Why is this any different from the workouts I've tried before?" Here's the scoop: isometric exercises aren't about endless repetitions or frenzied cardio sessions. They're about control, precision, and intentional muscle engagement. It's like the difference between a chaotic dance floor and a graceful ballet – both burn calories, but one sculpts with finesse.

Isometrics defy the norms of traditional workouts. No jumping, no running, just pure, intentional holds that target your muscles with surgical precision. It's like the difference between shouting in a crowded room and delivering a powerful speech that resonates. With isometrics, every second of stillness packs a punch, working your muscles in ways you never thought possible.

Let's get a bit nerdy for a moment, shall we? There's more to isometrics than meets the eye. The science behind it is fascinating – by engaging your muscles without movement, isometrics enhance blood flow, promote flexibility, and trigger the release of endorphins, your body's natural painkillers. It's not just a workout; it's a prescription for relief.

Think of it this way: imagine your muscles as a well-orchestrated symphony. Isometric exercises are the conductor, bringing each muscle into harmony, reducing tension, and soothing pain.

Chapter 2
Getting Started with Isometrics
Preparing for Your Isometric Journey

Welcome to the gateway of your isometric adventure! In this chapter, we're laying down the foundation for your journey into the world of static contractions. So, grab your metaphorical map and let's navigate the path to pain relief and strength together.

Before we dive into the exercises, it's crucial to set the stage for success. Think of it like preparing for a road trip – you wouldn't hit the highway without checking your car, right? Similarly, let's ensure you're equipped and ready for the isometric journey ahead.

1. Mindset Matters: Unlock Your Potential

Isometrics isn't just a physical workout; it's a mental game too. Embrace the mindset of intentional, focused effort. Visualize your muscles working, imagine the pain dissipating, and believe in the power of each isometric hold.

2. Space and Equipment: Create Your Workout Haven

The beauty of isometrics lies in its simplicity. You don't need fancy equipment or a sprawling gym. Find a quiet space where you can move freely without interruptions. A yoga mat or a comfortable carpet can be your workout haven.

3. Attire: Dress for Success

Think comfort and flexibility. Wear breathable clothing that allows for unrestricted movement. Isometric exercises involve holding positions, so comfort is key.

4. Hydration: Nourish Your Muscles

Hydrate before, during, and after your workout. Water is the fuel that keeps your muscles firing on all cylinders. Think of it as the refreshment station on your fitness journey.

5. Posture Check: Set the Foundation

Good posture is your secret weapon in isometrics. Align your body properly to engage the right muscles. Imagine your body as a well-stacked tower – strong, stable, and ready for action.

6. Warm-Up Ritual: Ignite Your Muscles

A dynamic warm-up primes your muscles for action. Incorporate light cardio, gentle stretches, and joint rotations to get the blood flowing. Think of it as tuning up your engine before a race.

7. Breathing Awareness: Oxygenate Your Efforts

Pay attention to your breath. Deep, controlled breathing not only fuels your muscles but also enhances focus. Inhale confidence, exhale doubt – it's your rhythm of empowerment.

Isometrics should challenge you, not hurt you. If you feel pain beyond the usual burn, reassess your form. Your body communicates – listen to it. This is a journey, not a sprint.

Now that we've prepped the canvas, it's time to paint the picture of your isometric journey. In the next chapters, we'll pick up the brushes and dive into specific exercises tailored for pain relief and strength. Ready to sculpt a masterpiece? The isometric canvas awaits!

Importance of Proper Form and Technique

As we embark on our isometric journey, consider this chapter as your compass and anchor. Here, we delve into the critical components of proper form and technique – the guiding principles that will not only maximize the benefits of your isometric exercises but also ensure your safety throughout the adventure.

Importance of Proper Form and Technique

Imagine you're crafting a delicate piece of art. Each stroke, each detail matters. Isometric exercises are no different. Proper form and technique are the brushes that sculpt your body with precision and finesse. Let's unravel the significance:

1. Muscle Targeting: Precision in Action

Proper form ensures that you're targeting the right muscles. Think of it like a laser beam – precise and effective. Whether it's your back, neck, or knees, the right form directs the effort where it matters most.

2. Optimizing Results: Quality Over Quantity

It's not about how many reps you can do; it's about the quality of each hold. Proper form maximizes the effectiveness of each isometric contraction, unlocking the full potential of your muscles.

3. Injury Prevention: Shielding Your Body

Think of your body as a temple. With the right form, you're not just exercising; you're protecting your joints, ligaments, and tendons from unnecessary strain. It's your shield against the risk of injury.

4. Posture Enhancement: Strength Beyond the Workout

Isometric exercises spill over into everyday life. The good posture you cultivate during isometrics becomes a habit, alleviating stress on your spine and enhancing your overall physical presence.

5. Mind-Body Connection: Harmony in Motion

Proper form isn't just a physical concept; it's a dance between your mind and body. It fosters a deeper connection, making each isometric hold a symphony of intention and strength.

Safety Considerations

Safety is our top priority on this journey. Isometric exercises are meant to challenge you, not harm you. Let's establish the safety guidelines that will be your steadfast companions:

1. Listen to Your Body: The Wisest Guide

Your body communicates with you. If an exercise causes pain beyond the usual burn, pause and reassess. It's okay to challenge yourself, but it's equally important to respect your body's signals.

2. Gradual Progression: Step by Step Mastery

Rome wasn't built in a day, and neither is your strength. Progress gradually. Begin with basic isometric holds, mastering each before progressing to more challenging exercises. It's a journey, not a race.

3. Warm-Up Ritual: Prep Your Muscles

We've touched on this before, but it's worth emphasizing. A proper warm-up isn't just a formality; it's a crucial step in preparing your muscles for the demands of isometric training.

4. Hydration: Sip Safely

Dehydration can compromise your performance and increase the risk of cramps. Keep sipping water throughout your workout, ensuring your body stays hydrated and ready for action.

Rest is as crucial as the workout itself. Allow your muscles time to recover. Overtraining can lead to fatigue and increased risk of injury.

Consider this chapter as your safety harness. As we progress into the specific isometric exercises in the following chapters, keep these principles in mind. Your journey is not just about reaching the destination; it's about savoring each step, sculpting your body with care, and embracing the empowerment that isometrics bring. Onward, fellow adventurer!

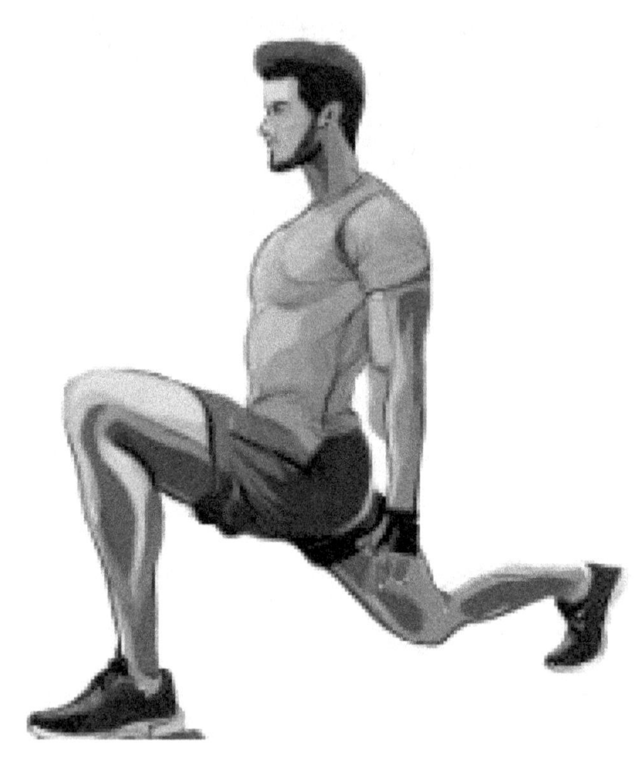

Chapter 3
Targeting Common Aches and Pains
Relieving Back Pain with Isometrics

Welcome to the heart of our isometric journey! In this chapter, we hone in on a prevalent adversary – back pain. Whether it's a dull ache or a persistent discomfort, we're about to explore how isometric exercises can be your ally in finding relief. So, roll out your metaphorical yoga mat, and let's dive into the art of alleviating back pain through isometrics.

Picture your back as the sturdy foundation of a skyscraper. It bears the weight of your world, and when it protests, everything feels a bit shaky. Isometric exercises, however, offer a unique solution – a way to strengthen and stabilize your back muscles without putting undue stress on the spine. Let's embark on a step-by-step journey to alleviate back pain:

1. Find Your Comfort Zone:

Start by finding a quiet space where you can lay down on your back. Use a yoga mat or a comfortable surface.

2. The Foundation: Neutral Spine Position:

Lie down with your back on the mat, knees bent, and feet flat on the ground. Ensure your spine is in a neutral position – not overly arched or flattened against the mat.

3. Engage Your Core: The Powerhouse:

Before we dive into specific isometric holds, engage your core. Imagine pulling your belly button towards your spine. This creates a stable foundation for the exercises.

4. Isometric Hold 1: Bridge Pose - Strength and Stability:

Lift your hips towards the ceiling, creating a straight line from your shoulders to your knees. Hold this position for 20-30 seconds, focusing on the contraction in your glutes and lower back. Breathe steadily throughout.

5. Rest and Reset: Neutral Position:

Lower your hips back down, rest for a moment in the neutral position, and reassess how your back feels.

6. Isometric Hold 2: Superman Pose - Targeting Lower Back:

Extend your arms forward and lift your right arm and left leg off the ground simultaneously. Hold for 15-20 seconds, feeling the engagement in your lower back and opposite glute. Switch sides and repeat.

7. Rest and Reset: Neutral Position:

Return to the neutral position, allowing your spine to relax for a brief moment.

8. Isometric Hold 3: Side Plank - Core and Lateral Muscles:

Shift onto your side, supporting your body on your elbow and side of the foot. Lift your hips, creating a straight line from head to toe. Hold for 20-30 seconds on each side, feeling the activation in your lateral muscles.

End your back pain relief routine with Savasana. Lie on your back, arms by your sides, and let your body sink into the mat. Focus on your breath and allow any remaining tension to melt away.

This sequence of isometric exercises is designed to target different muscle groups in your back, providing relief and strengthening the supporting structures. As you embrace each hold, listen to your body, and modify as needed. Consistency is the key on this journey, and with each session, you're sculpting a stronger, more resilient back.

In the following chapters, we'll continue our exploration,* addressing neck pain, knee discomfort, and muscle soreness across the body. The isometric canvas is vast, and the relief it brings is profound. Until then, revel in the newfound strength and comfort of your back – a testament to the power of isometrics. Onward to pain-free living!

Alleviating Neck and Shoulder Tension

Welcome to the next phase of our isometric journey!* In this chapter, we turn our attention to a common source of discomfort, neck and shoulder tension. The demands of modern life often leave these areas vulnerable to stress and strain. Fear not, as we explore isometric exercises specifically tailored to provide relief and release the tension that may have nestled itself in your neck and shoulders. So, find a quiet space, roll out that metaphorical yoga mat, and let's delve into the art of alleviating neck and shoulder tension through isometrics.

Alleviating Neck and Shoulder Tension

Your neck and shoulders are the bridge between your head and body. When tension sets in, it's as if that bridge is under construction not the smoothest journey. Isometric exercises offer a therapeutic approach, targeting these areas with precision. Let's embark on a step-by-step guide to alleviate neck and shoulder tension:

1. Set the Scene: Find a Comfortable Position:

Sit or stand comfortably in a quiet space. Relax your shoulders and let your arms rest naturally by your sides.

2. Chin Tucks: Nurturing the Neck:

Begin by gently tucking your chin towards your chest, creating a subtle stretch along the back of your neck. Hold this position for 15-20 seconds, feeling the release in the cervical spine.

3. Ear-to-Shoulder Stretch: Easing Shoulder Tension:

Slowly tilt your head to one side, bringing your ear towards your shoulder. Hold for 15-20 seconds, allowing the stretch to alleviate tension along the side of your neck and shoulder. Repeat on the other side.

4. Isometric Hold 1: Neck Resistance - Frontal Tension Release:

Place your hand against your forehead, and gently press your head forward while resisting with your neck muscles. Hold for 10-15 seconds, feeling the engagement in the front of your neck. Release and repeat.

5. Isometric Hold 2: Shoulder Shrug - Elevating and Relaxing:

Lift your shoulders towards your ears, creating tension in the upper trapezius muscles. Hold for 15-20 seconds, then consciously relax your shoulders down. Repeat this shrugging motion several times.

6. Isometric Hold 3: Side Neck Resistance - Lateral Release:

Place your hand on the side of your head and gently press, tilting your head towards the opposite shoulder while resisting with your neck muscles. Hold for 10-15 seconds, feeling the lateral stretch. Release and switch sides.

7. Final Relaxation: Neck and Shoulder Rolls - Unwind and Release:

Sit or stand comfortably, and gently roll your shoulders in circular motions, both clockwise and counterclockwise. This fluid motion helps release any remaining tension in your neck and shoulders.

Remember, the key is to move slowly and deliberately, allowing the isometric holds to target specific muscle groups. Each movement is a conscious effort to release tension and promote relaxation. Listen to your body, and modify the intensity as needed.

As we progress on our isometric journey, the next chapters will address knee discomfort and muscle soreness across the body. You're not just relieving tension; you're fostering a sense of ease and freedom in your body. Enjoy the newfound lightness in your neck and shoulders – a testament to the power of isometrics. Onward to a more relaxed and pain-free you!

Isometric Solutions for Knee Discomfort

Welcome to the chapter designed to bring relief to a common source of discomfort – knee pain. Whether it's a twinge, a persistent ache, or discomfort during movement, your knees deserve special attention. In this segment of our isometric journey, we'll explore targeted exercises crafted to strengthen and stabilize the muscles around your knees, providing solutions for knee discomfort. So, find a comfortable space, gather your metaphorical equipment, and let's delve into the art of addressing knee discomfort through isometrics.

Isometric Solutions for Knee Discomfort

Your knees are intricate joints, often bearing the brunt of daily activities.* When discomfort sets in, it can impact your mobility and overall well-being. Isometric exercises offer a unique approach, honing in on the muscles that support and protect the knee joint.

1. Starting Position: Stand Tall and Align:

Begin by standing tall with your feet hip-width apart. Ensure your weight is evenly distributed between both legs, and your knees are in a relaxed, slightly bent position.

2. Isometric Hold 1: Quad Contractions - Strengthening the Front Muscles:

Lift one foot slightly off the ground and engage your quadriceps by straightening your lifted leg. Hold for 10-15 seconds, feeling the contraction in the front of your thigh. Switch legs and repeat.

3. Isometric Hold 2: Hamstring Contractions - Strengthening the Back Muscles:

Stand with your feet hip-width apart. Shift your weight to one leg and slightly lift the other foot off the ground. Engage your hamstrings by bending your lifted leg at the knee. Hold for 10-15 seconds, feeling the engagement in the back of your thigh. Switch legs and repeat.

4. Isometric Hold 3: Inner Thigh Squeeze - Strengthening Medial Muscles:

Place a soft ball or cushion between your knees. Squeeze the ball gently with your inner thighs, engaging the muscles on the inside of your leg. Hold for 15-20 seconds and release.

5. Isometric Hold 4: Outer Thigh Push - Strengthening Lateral Muscles:

Place a resistance band around your ankles. Step to the side against the band's resistance, engaging the muscles on the outside of your leg. Hold for 15-20 seconds and return to the starting position. Repeat on the other side.

6. Full Range Leg Lifts: Controlled Movement for Stability:

- Stand near a sturdy surface for support. Lift one leg forward, then to the side, and finally to the back, moving through the full range of motion. Perform 10 repetitions on each leg, ensuring controlled movements.

Sit on the floor with your legs extended in front of you. Bend one knee and bring the sole of your foot against the inner thigh of the opposite leg. Gently lean forward to feel a stretch in the back of the extended leg. Hold for 20-30 seconds and switch sides.

These isometric exercises are designed to target different muscle groups around your knees, offering support, strength, and relief from discomfort. Remember to perform each movement slowly and deliberately, focusing on the engagement of specific muscle groups.

As we continue our isometric journey, the next chapters will address other common areas of discomfort and muscle soreness across the body. With each exercise, you're not just addressing knee discomfort; you're building a foundation of strength and resilience. Onward to a more stable and pain-free you!

Addressing Muscle Soreness Across the Body

Welcome to the comprehensive segment of our isometric journey! In this chapter, we'll explore the holistic approach of isometric exercises to address muscle soreness across various parts of the body. Whether it's aching muscles from a workout, stiffness from a long day, or general soreness that lingers, these exercises are tailored to provide relief and foster overall muscle well-being. So, prepare your metaphorical workout space, and let's delve into the art of addressing muscle soreness across the body through isometrics.

Muscle soreness is a universal experience, and addressing it comprehensively involves engaging various muscle groups. Isometric exercises provide a unique solution, targeting sore areas and promoting overall muscle recovery. Let's explore a series of exercises designed to address muscle soreness across the body:

1. Starting Position: Stand or Sit Comfortably:

Begin in a comfortable standing or sitting position. Take a moment to center yourself, focusing on your breath.

2. Isometric Hold 1: Full-Body Tension Release - Progressive Muscle Relaxation:

Start from your toes and work your way up, progressively tensing and then releasing each muscle group. Begin with your toes, move to your calves, thighs, and continue upward through your torso, arms, and neck. This exercise helps release tension and promote overall relaxation.

3. Isometric Hold 2: Dynamic Arm Circles - Mobilizing the Upper Body:

Extend your arms to the sides and make small, controlled circles in both directions. Gradually increase the size of the circles, engaging your shoulder muscles. Perform this movement for 1-2 minutes to enhance blood flow and reduce stiffness.

4. Isometric Hold 3: Seated Leg Lifts - Engaging Lower Body Muscles:

Sit on a chair with your feet flat on the ground. Lift one leg at a time, engaging your thigh muscles. Hold each lift for 10-15 seconds, alternating between legs. This exercise helps activate and relieve tension in the lower body.

5. Isometric Hold 4: Dynamic Torso Twists - Mobilizing the Core:

Stand with your feet hip-width apart. Twist your torso to one side, then the other, in a controlled and dynamic motion. Engage your core muscles as you twist. Perform for 1-2 minutes to promote flexibility and alleviate soreness in the torso.

6. Isometric Hold 5: Neck and Shoulder Stretch - Relaxing Upper Body Muscles:

Gently tilt your head to one side, bringing your ear towards your shoulder. Hold for 15-20 seconds, feeling the stretch along the side of your neck and shoulder. Repeat on the other side.

7. Full-Body Stretch: Cat-Cow Stretch - Dynamic Spinal Release:

Start on your hands and knees. Inhale as you arch your back, dropping your belly towards the ground (Cow). Exhale as you round your back, tucking your chin to your chest (Cat). Repeat this dynamic stretch for 1-2 minutes to release tension along the spine.

8. Final Relaxation: Corpse Pose (Savasana) - Complete Muscle Relaxation:

Lie down on your back, arms by your sides, and let your body sink into the floor. Focus on your breath and allow any remaining tension to dissipate. Hold this relaxation pose for 5-10 minutes.

These isometric exercises are designed to provide a comprehensive approach to addressing muscle soreness,* promoting flexibility, and enhancing overall well-being. Perform each exercise mindfully, paying attention to the engagement of specific muscle groups.

As we continue our isometric journey, the following chapters will delve deeper into advanced techniques and explore the integration of isometrics with dynamic movements. Each exercise is a step toward not only addressing muscle soreness but also building a foundation of strength and flexibility. Onward to a rejuvenated and invigorated you!

Chapter 4
Isometric Routines for Joint Health
Improving Joint Flexibility and Strength

Welcome to the pivotal chapter dedicated to enhancing the health of your joints through purposeful isometric routines!* In this segment of our isometric journey, we'll focus on the delicate balance of improving joint flexibility and strength. Joints are the unsung heroes of movement, and with targeted isometric exercises, we aim to fortify their resilience and enhance their range of motion. So, prepare your metaphorical workout space, and let's delve into the art of fostering joint health through isometrics.

Improving Joint Flexibility and Strength

Your joints are the hinges of your body, facilitating every movement, bend, and twist. As we age or engage in repetitive activities, joints can become stiff, limiting our range of motion and causing discomfort. Isometric exercises offer a strategic approach, combining strength-building with flexibility enhancement to promote overall joint health. Let's navigate through a series of exercises designed to improve joint flexibility and strength:

1. Starting Position: Sit or Stand with Mindful Posture:

Begin in a comfortable seated or standing position. Ensure your spine is aligned, and your shoulders are relaxed. Take a few deep breaths to center yourself.

2. Isometric Hold 1: Neck Nods - Gentle Neck Flexibility:

Slowly nod your head forward, bringing your chin towards your chest. Hold for 10-15 seconds, feeling the stretch along the back of your neck. Return to the neutral position and repeat.

3. Isometric Hold 2: Wrist Contractions - Strengthening the Wrists:

Extend your arms in front of you at shoulder height. Make a fist with each hand and engage your wrist muscles by pressing your fists against each other. Hold for 10-15 seconds and release. Repeat.

4. Isometric Hold 3: Seated Knee Press - Strengthening Knee Joints:

Sit on a chair with your feet flat on the ground. Place your hands on your knees and press them against each other, engaging the muscles around your knee joints. Hold for 15-20 seconds and release.

5. Isometric Hold 4: Hip Abduction - Strengthening Hips:

Stand with your feet hip-width apart. Lift one leg to the side, engaging the muscles on the outer hip. Hold for 15-20 seconds and return to the starting position. Repeat on the other leg.

6. Isometric Hold 5: Ankle Circles - Improving Ankle Flexibility:

Sit on the floor with your legs extended. Lift one foot off the ground and make slow circles with your ankle in both directions. Perform for 1-2 minutes and switch to the other foot.

7. *Full-Body Stretch: Forward Bend - Dynamic Spinal Flexibility:*

Stand with your feet hip-width apart. Slowly hinge at your hips, reaching towards the ground. Allow your spine to lengthen as you stretch forward. Hold for 15-20 seconds and return to the upright position.

8. *Isometric Hold 6: Shoulder Blade Squeeze - Enhancing Shoulder Mobility:*

Stand or sit comfortably. Squeeze your shoulder blades together, as if trying to hold a pencil between them. Hold for 10-15 seconds and release. Repeat.

9. *Final Relaxation: Child's Pose - Total Body Release:*

Kneel on the floor with your toes together and knees apart. Sit back on your heels and extend your arms forward. Rest your forehead on the ground and hold for 5-10 breaths.

These isometric routines are tailored to enhance joint flexibility and strength, addressing various joints throughout the body. Perform each exercise with mindful engagement, focusing on the targeted muscles and joints.

As we progress through our isometric journey, the subsequent chapters will explore advanced techniques and integrative routines to elevate your joint health and overall physical well-being. Each exercise is a step towards not only improving joint flexibility and strength but also fostering a sense of balance and harmony within your body. Onward to resilient and flexible joints!

Isometric Exercises for Arthritis Relief

Welcome to a crucial chapter focused on providing relief for arthritis through purposeful isometric exercises!* In this segment of our isometric journey, we'll address the unique challenges posed by arthritis and explore exercises designed to alleviate discomfort and enhance joint function. Moreover, we'll delve into the proactive approach of preventing joint injuries through regular isometrics. So, find a comfortable space, and let's navigate through the art of promoting arthritis relief and preventing joint injuries with isometrics.

Arthritis, with its inflammation and stiffness, demands a thoughtful and gentle approach. Isometric exercises offer a tailored solution, providing relief for arthritis symptoms without placing excessive strain on the joints. Let's explore a series of exercises designed to alleviate arthritis discomfort:

1. Starting Position: Find a Comfortable Seated or Standing Stance:

Begin in a comfortable seated or standing position. Take a moment to relax your shoulders and center yourself.

2. Isometric Hold 1: Gentle Neck Rotation - Easing Neck Discomfort:

Slowly turn your head to one side, holding the position for 10-15 seconds. Feel the gentle stretch in your neck. Return to the center and repeat on the other side.

3. Isometric Hold 2: Hand Grip Strengthener - Relieving Hand Arthritis:

Extend your fingers and make a fist, holding for 10-15 seconds. Release and spread your fingers wide, holding again. This exercise helps alleviate stiffness and enhances hand flexibility.

4. Isometric Hold 3: Seated Leg Press - Strengthening Knee Joints:

Sit on a chair with your feet flat on the ground. Press your knees together, engaging the muscles around your knee joints. Hold for 15-20 seconds and release.

5. Isometric Hold 4: Hip Flexor Engagement - Easing Hip Discomfort:

Stand with your feet hip-width apart. Lift one knee towards your chest, engaging your hip flexors. Hold for 10-15 seconds and lower your leg. Repeat on the other side.

6. Isometric Hold 5: Wall Push-Up - Supporting Elbows and Shoulders:

Stand facing a wall with your palms against it. Press your palms into the wall, engaging your elbows and shoulders. Hold for 15-20 seconds and release.

7. Isometric Hold 6: Seated Heel Raises - Ankle Mobility Enhancement:

Sit on a chair with your feet flat on the ground. Lift your heels off the floor, engaging your calf muscles. Hold for 10-15 seconds and lower your heels.

8. Isometric Hold 7: Gentle Torso Twist - Promoting Spinal Flexibility:

Sit or stand comfortably. Slowly twist your torso to one side, holding for 10-15 seconds. Feel the gentle stretch along your spine. Return to the center and repeat on the other side.

Preventing Joint Injuries with Regular Isometrics

Prevention is a powerful aspect of joint care, especially for individuals with arthritis. Regular isometric exercises can be a proactive measure to safeguard joint health and minimize the risk of injuries. Let's explore guidelines for integrating regular isometrics into your routine:

1. Consistency is Key:

Incorporate isometric exercises into your routine regularly. Consistency is vital for maintaining joint flexibility and strength.

2. Gradual Progression:

Start with gentle exercises and gradually progress to more challenging ones. Listen to your body and tailor the intensity to your comfort level.

3. Balance with Rest:

Balance your isometric exercises with proper rest. Allow your joints to recover, especially if you experience any discomfort.

4. Mindful Movement:

Practice each isometric exercise with mindfulness. Pay attention to the sensations in your joints and modify movements if needed.

5. Consultation with Healthcare Provider:

Before starting any new exercise regimen, especially for individuals with arthritis, consult with your healthcare provider.

They can provide personalized guidance based on your specific condition.

As we continue our isometric journey, the subsequent chapters will delve into additional techniques and integrative routines to further enhance joint health and overall well-being. Each exercise is a step towards not only relieving arthritis symptoms but also promoting a proactive approach to joint care. Onward to a more comfortable and resilient you!

Chapter 5
Customizing Your Isometric Workout
Tailoring Exercises to Your Fitness Level

Welcome to a pivotal chapter that empowers you to customize your isometric workout according to your unique fitness level! In this segment of our isometric journey, we'll explore the flexibility and adaptability of isometric exercises, allowing you to tailor your workout to suit your current fitness capabilities. Whether you're a beginner seeking a gentle introduction or an experienced fitness enthusiast looking for a challenge, this chapter will guide you in crafting a workout that aligns with your individual needs. So, find a comfortable space, and let's dive into the art of customizing your isometric workout.

The beauty of isometric exercises lies in their versatility; they can be modified to accommodate various fitness levels. Whether you're a newcomer to the world of isometrics or a seasoned practitioner, customizing your workout ensures a personalized and effective fitness experience. Let's explore how you can adapt isometric exercises to match your fitness level:

1. Assess Your Fitness Level:

Begin by honestly assessing your current fitness level. Consider your strength, flexibility, and any physical limitations. This self-awareness forms the foundation for customization.!

2. *Start with Fundamentals:*

If you're new to isometrics or returning after a break, start with fundamental exercises. Focus on mastering basic holds and gentle movements to build a solid foundation.

3. *Modify Intensity:*

Isometric exercises can be easily modified by adjusting the intensity. For beginners, start with shorter hold times and gradually increase as your strength improves. For advanced practitioners, extend hold times or add resistance for an extra challenge.

4. *Choose Appropriate Exercises:*

Select exercises that align with your current fitness level and goals. Beginners may choose simpler movements targeting major muscle groups, while advanced individuals can explore complex holds and dynamic isometric sequences.

5. *Include Progressive Challenges:*

As your fitness progresses, incorporate progressive challenges. This could involve adding resistance, increasing hold times, or exploring advanced variations of familiar exercises. Progressive challenges keep your workout dynamic and stimulating.

6. *Listen to Your Body:*

Pay attention to how your body responds to each exercise. If you experience pain or discomfort beyond normal muscle fatigue, consider modifying the movement or seeking guidance from a fitness professional.

7. Include Rest and Recovery:

Regardless of your fitness level, adequate rest and recovery are essential. Allow your muscles and joints time to recover between workouts to prevent overtraining and promote long-term sustainability.

8. Incorporate Variety:

Keep your workout engaging by incorporating a variety of isometric exercises. This not only targets different muscle groups but also adds an element of excitement to your routine.

Sample Customized Isometric Workout:

Beginner's Routine:

1. Basic Wall Sit - 3 sets of 15 seconds
2. Seated Leg Press - 2 sets of 12 repetitions
3. Wrist Contractions - 2 sets of 15 seconds
4. Chest Press against a Wall - 3 sets of 10 seconds
5. Standing Calf Raise Hold - 2 sets of 20 seconds

Advanced Routine:

1. Advanced Plank - 3 sets of 30 seconds
2. Single-Leg Squat Hold - 2 sets of 20 seconds per leg
3. Handstand against a Wall - 3 sets of 20 seconds
4. Isometric Pull-Ups - 2 sets of 10 seconds
5. Lateral Leg Raise Hold - 2 sets of 25 seconds per side

Remember, the key is to customize your workout based on your individual needs, gradually progressing as your fitness level improves.

Incorporating Isometrics into Your Existing Routine

Welcome to a dynamic chapter that explores the seamless integration of isometrics into your existing fitness routine, tailored for different age groups! In this segment of our isometric journey, we'll delve into the versatility of isometric exercises, providing insights on how to blend them with your current workout regimen. Additionally, we'll discuss the adaptability of isometrics, ensuring they cater to the unique needs and abilities of various age groups. So, find your comfortable workout space, and let's explore the art of incorporating isometrics into your routine for a well-rounded fitness experience.

Whether you're a seasoned fitness enthusiast or someone just beginning their fitness journey, isometrics can seamlessly complement your existing routine, adding a layer of depth and effectiveness.

1. Warm-Up with Isometric Holds:

Begin your workout with isometric holds to activate and engage major muscle groups. This helps prepare your body for more dynamic movements and reduces the risk of injury.

2. Integrate Isometric Holds Between Sets:

Enhance the intensity of your strength training routine by incorporating isometric holds between sets. For example, perform a wall sit or plank for 20-30 seconds before moving on to the next set of exercises.

3. Replace Dynamic Exercises with Isometric Variations:

Experiment with replacing some dynamic exercises with their isometric variations. For instance, replace traditional squats with a static squat hold against a wall to intensify the muscle engagement.

4. Cool Down with Relaxing Isometric Stretches:

Conclude your workout with isometric stretches to improve flexibility and promote relaxation. These static stretches help release tension in muscles worked during the workout.

5. Combine Isometrics with Cardiovascular Exercise:

For those engaged in cardiovascular activities like running or cycling, incorporate isometric exercises during intervals. For example, perform standing calf raises during a jogging break to strengthen your calf muscles.

6. Adapt Isometrics for Home Workouts:

If you prefer working out at home, isometrics are ideal. Exercises like wall sits, plank variations, and isometric lunges require minimal space and no equipment, making them perfect for home workouts.

Adapting Isometrics for Different Age Groups

Isometrics are versatile and can be adapted to cater to the specific needs and capabilities of different age groups.* Whether you're a young adult, middle-aged, or a senior, consider the following guidelines for incorporating isometrics into your fitness routine:

1. Young Adults (18-35):

Young adults can explore a wide range of dynamic and challenging isometric exercises. Incorporate explosive isometric movements like squat jumps or advanced plank variations for strength and endurance.

2. Middle-Aged Adults (36-60):

Focus on a balanced approach that addresses strength, flexibility, and joint health. Include isometric exercises that target the core, hips, and shoulders to maintain functional fitness.

3. Seniors (60 and above):

Prioritize safety and joint health. Choose low-impact isometric exercises such as seated leg lifts, wall push-ups, and gentle neck stretches. Emphasize stability and balance.

Sample Isometric Integration for Different Age Groups:

Young Adult Routine:

1. Explosive Wall Push-Ups - 3 sets of 15 reps
2. Dynamic Plank to Push-Up - 2 sets of 10 reps
3. Isometric Lunges - 3 sets of 20 seconds per leg
4. Standing Calf Raises with Pulse - 2 sets of 15 reps
5. Static Squat Hold - 2 sets of 30 seconds

Middle-Aged Adult Routine:

1. Plank with Shoulder Taps - 3 sets of 20 reps
2. Isometric Shoulder Press - 2 sets of 15 seconds
3. Seated Leg Press - 3 sets of 15 reps
4. Isometric Tricep Dips - 2 sets of 20 seconds
5. Wall Sit with Bicep Curl - 2 sets of 30 seconds

Senior Routine:

1. Seated Chest Press - 3 sets of 12 reps
2. Gentle Neck Stretch Hold - 2 sets of 20 seconds
3. Seated Leg Lifts - 3 sets of 15 reps
4. Wall Push-Ups with Hold - 2 sets of 15 seconds
5. Standing Balance Hold - 2 sets of 30 seconds

Remember, the key is to customize the intensity and complexity of isometric exercises based on individual fitness levels and goals. Whether you're aiming for strength, flexibility, or joint health, isometrics can be tailored to suit your needs.

As we advance in our isometric journey, subsequent chapters will explore specialized techniques and integrative routines for a well-rounded fitness experience. Onward to a versatile and adaptable approach to fitness!

Chapter 6
Advanced Isometric Techniques
Progressive Static Holds for Increased Strength

Welcome to a pivotal chapter that delves into the realm of advanced isometric techniques, designed to elevate your strength and endurance through strategic and progressive static holds. In this segment of our isometric journey, we'll explore techniques that go beyond the basics, challenging your muscles in new ways to unlock greater strength gains. So, prepare for a dynamic workout experience as we dive into the art of progressive static holds for increased strength.

As your fitness journey evolves, so should your approach to isometrics. Advanced techniques, particularly progressive static holds, are a powerful way to push your strength boundaries and stimulate muscle growth. Let's explore how you can incorporate these techniques into your routine:

1. Understanding Progressive Static Holds:

Progressive static holds involve gradually increasing the intensity or duration of a static hold over time. This progression challenges your muscles to adapt and grow stronger.

2. Selecting Appropriate Exercises:

Choose compound exercises that engage multiple muscle groups for maximum effectiveness. Examples include plank variations, wall sits, and isometric lunges.

3. Establishing Baseline Hold Times:

Begin with a baseline hold time that challenges you but allows for proper form. This could range from 10 to 30 seconds, depending on your current fitness level.

4. Increasing Duration Gradually:

Gradually increase the hold duration over successive sessions. Aim for small increments, such as adding 5 seconds per session. This gradual progression prevents overtraining and minimizes the risk of injury.

5. Incorporating Intensity Variations:

Introduce intensity variations to progressive static holds. This can involve adding resistance, changing body positions, or exploring advanced variations of the chosen exercise.

6. Maintaining Proper Form:

Focus on maintaining proper form throughout the hold. Sacrificing form for longer durations can lead to muscle imbalances and increased injury risk. Quality always trumps quantity.

Keep a workout journal to track your progress. Note the duration of each hold, any variations introduced, and how your body responds. This tracking helps you identify patterns and adjust your approach accordingly.

8. Sample Advanced Isometric Routine:

Week 1-2: Plank Hold - 3 sets of 20 seconds
Week 3-4: Plank Hold with Leg Lifts - 3 sets of 25 seconds
Week 5-6: Plank Hold with Alternating Arm and Leg Lifts - 3 sets of 30 seconds
Week 7-8: Plank Hold with Stability Ball - 3 sets of 35 seconds
Week 9-10: Plank Hold with Weighted Vest - 3 sets of 40 seconds

Benefits of Progressive Static Holds:

1. Muscle Engagement and Activation:

Progressive static holds force your muscles to remain engaged for extended periods, maximizing muscle activation and recruitment.

2. Strength Development:

By gradually increasing the intensity of static holds, you stimulate continuous strength development, promoting muscle hypertrophy and endurance.

3. Mental Resilience:

Pushing through progressively longer holds builds mental resilience and discipline, essential elements for achieving advanced fitness goals.

4. Joint Stability:

Isometric holds contribute to joint stability, reducing the risk of injuries during dynamic movements.

5. Time-Efficient Workouts:

Progressive static holds offer a time-efficient workout option, allowing you to target multiple muscle groups in a single exercise.

Safety Considerations:

- Ensure you have mastered basic isometric exercises before attempting progressive static holds.
- Listen to your body and avoid pushing beyond your limits to prevent injury.
- If you have any pre-existing conditions or concerns, consult with a fitness professional or healthcare provider before incorporating advanced techniques.

As we progress through our isometric journey,* subsequent chapters will explore additional advanced techniques and integrative routines to further enhance your strength, endurance, and overall fitness. Onward to the next level of strength gains and physical excellence!

Isometric Contractions for Muscle Endurance

Welcome to a transformative chapter that explores the synergy of isometric contractions and dynamic movements,* strategically combined to enhance muscle endurance and elevate your overall fitness experience. In this segment of our isometric journey, we'll delve into the dual benefits of isometrics and dynamic exercises, unlocking a new dimension of endurance and strength. So, let's embark on the art of combining isometric contractions with dynamic movements for a comprehensive and effective workout.

Isometric Contractions for Muscle Endurance

Isometric contractions are a cornerstone of muscle endurance training, providing a unique challenge by engaging muscles without lengthening or shortening them. When integrated into a workout routine, isometric contractions can significantly contribute to enhancing muscular endurance. Let's explore the principles and benefits:

1. Understanding Isometric Contractions:

Isometric contractions involve activating muscles without changing their length. Common examples include static holds, wall sits, or planks, where the muscle remains contracted for a specific duration.

Targeted Muscle Engagement: Isometrics activate specific muscle groups for an extended period, promoting endurance in those areas.

Joint Stability: Isometric contractions enhance joint stability, reducing the risk of injuries during prolonged or repetitive movements.

Mental Endurance: Holding a static position builds mental endurance, helping you push through fatigue and maintain focus.

3. Sample Isometric Endurance Routine:

Wall Sit: 3 sets of 45 seconds
Plank: 3 sets of 1 minute
Isometric Squat Hold: 3 sets of 30 seconds
Static Lunge: 3 sets of 40 seconds per leg

Combining Isometrics with Dynamic Movements

The synergy of isometrics with dynamic movements creates a comprehensive and challenging workout experience. By seamlessly integrating these two approaches, you engage muscles in various ways, fostering strength, flexibility, and endurance. Let's explore how to combine isometrics with dynamic exercises:

1. Isometric-Dynamic Supersets:

Pair an isometric exercise with a dynamic movement in a superset fashion. For example, combine a plank hold with mountain climbers. This challenges your muscles with both static endurance and dynamic engagement.

2. Transitioning from Isometric to Dynamic:

Start with an isometric hold and seamlessly transition into a dynamic movement targeting the same muscle group. For instance, perform a wall sit and then progress into bodyweight squats. This transition challenges muscles to adapt quickly.

3. Isometric Holds within Dynamic Sequences:

Incorporate brief isometric holds within dynamic exercise sequences. For example, during a set of lunges, pause at the lowest point of the movement for a 10-second isometric hold before transitioning to the next lunge.

4. Dynamic Movements Between Isometric Holds:

Introduce dynamic movements between isometric holds. For instance, perform a set of isometric push-ups followed by explosive plyometric push-ups. This combination targets both strength and power.

5. Example Isometric-Dynamic Workout:

Superset 1:
 - Isometric Squat Hold - 3 sets of 30 seconds
 - Bodyweight Squats - 3 sets of 15 reps
Superset 2:
 - Plank with Shoulder Taps - 3 sets of 45 seconds
 - Mountain Climbers - 3 sets of 20 reps
Superset 3:
 - Wall Sit - 3 sets of 40 seconds
 - Jumping Lunges - 3 sets of 15 reps per leg

Benefits of Combining Isometrics with Dynamic Movements:

1. Enhanced Muscle Recruitment:

The combination challenges muscles in multiple ways, promoting comprehensive muscle recruitment and development.

2. Improved Cardiovascular Endurance:

Dynamic movements elevate the heart rate, contributing to improved cardiovascular endurance when paired with isometric holds.

3. Functional Strength Development:

The integration of dynamic movements enhances functional strength, translating to improved performance in daily activities and sports.

4. Caloric Expenditure:

The dynamic component increases caloric expenditure, making the workout effective for those seeking both endurance and calorie burn.

5. Versatility and Engagement:

The variety of movements keeps the workout engaging, reducing monotony and enhancing overall workout enjoyment.

Safety Considerations:
- Pay attention to proper form during dynamic movements to avoid injury.
- Gradually increase intensity to allow your body to adapt to the combination of isometrics and dynamic exercises.
- Listen to your body and modify movements if needed, especially if you have pre-existing conditions.

As we progress further in our isometric journey, subsequent chapters will explore advanced techniques and specialized routines to continue elevating your fitness experience. Onward to the dynamic fusion of isometrics and dynamic movements for enduring strength and vitality!

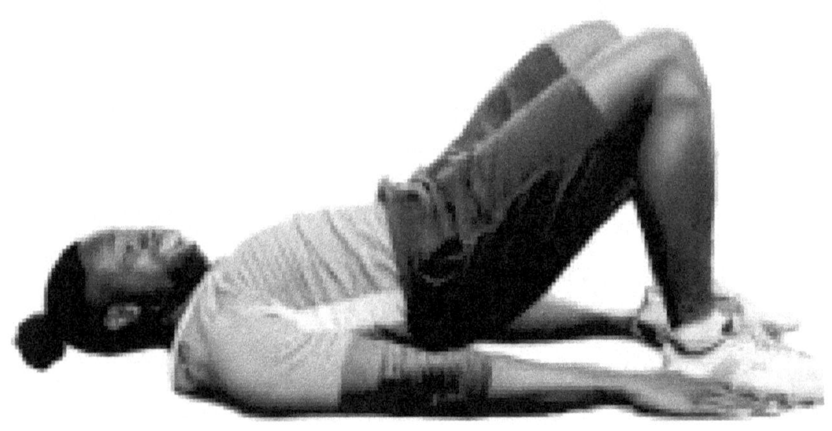

Chapter 7
Mind-Body Connection in Isometric Training
Incorporating Mindfulness and Breathing Techniques

Welcome to a transformative chapter that delves into the powerful connection between the mind and body* in the realm of isometric training. In this segment of our isometric journey, we'll explore how mindfulness and intentional breathing techniques can enhance the effectiveness of isometric exercises. Additionally, we'll uncover the profound impact isometrics can have on stress reduction, offering a holistic approach to both physical and mental well-being.

The mind-body connection is a cornerstone of holistic well-being. Integrating mindfulness and intentional breathing into your isometric training not only deepens your awareness of physical sensations but also contributes to a more focused and centered workout experience. Let's explore how to infuse mindfulness and breathing techniques into your isometric routine:

1. Mindful Awareness of Muscle Engagement:

Before initiating an isometric hold, take a moment to bring awareness to the specific muscles you'll be engaging. This mindful approach enhances the neural connection between your brain and muscles, optimizing their activation.

2. Conscious Breath Alignment:

Align your breath with the isometric contraction. Inhale deeply before initiating the hold, and exhale slowly as you sustain the static position. Conscious breathing promotes relaxation, reduces tension, and improves overall endurance.

3. Focused Attention on Sensations:

Throughout the isometric hold, maintain a focused attention on the sensations within your body. Notice the subtle shifts, muscle engagement, and areas of tension or release. This heightened awareness deepens the mind-body connection.

4. Guided Meditation during Isometrics:

Consider incorporating short guided meditations during isometric holds. Focus on positive affirmations, gratitude, or visualization to create a positive mental environment during your workout.

5. Breathing Techniques for Intensity Control:

Experiment with different breathing patterns to modulate the intensity of isometric holds. Slow, controlled breaths can enhance stability, while more rapid breaths may support explosive or dynamic isometric movements.

6. Post-Isometric Relaxation:

After completing an isometric hold, take a moment for intentional relaxation. Release tension in the muscles, and focus on slow, calming breaths to transition smoothly to the next exercise.

Enhancing Stress Reduction through Isometrics

Isometric exercises offer more than just physical benefits; they can be powerful tools for stress reduction.* The intentional focus required during isometric holds, combined with controlled breathing, creates a calming effect on the nervous system. Let's explore how isometrics can be harnessed to enhance stress reduction:

1. Isometrics as Mindful Pause:

Isometric exercises serve as mindful pauses in your day. Taking a break to engage in a brief isometric hold redirects your attention away from stressors, allowing a mental reset.

2. Tension Release through Static Holds:

The deliberate engagement and subsequent release of muscles during isometric holds can serve as a cathartic experience, helping release physical tension associated with stress.

3. Cortisol Regulation with Isometrics:

Regular practice of isometrics has been linked to cortisol regulation, the stress hormone. By managing cortisol levels through exercise, you contribute to overall stress resilience.

4. Mindfulness in Stressful Situations:

The mindfulness cultivated during isometric training extends beyond the workout. You'll find yourself better equipped to maintain a calm and focused mindset during daily stressors.

5. Stress-Relief Isometric Routine:

Create a short routine focusing on stress-relief isometric exercises, such as seated meditation holds, gentle stretches, and controlled breathing. This routine can serve as a quick and effective stress-buster.

Benefits of Mind-Body Connection in Isometric Training:

1. Improved Focus and Concentration:

Mindfulness enhances your ability to stay present during isometric exercises, promoting improved focus and concentration.

2. Heightened Body Awareness:

Mindful awareness of muscle engagement and breathing patterns cultivates a heightened sense of body awareness, contributing to better form and control.

3. Stress Reduction and Relaxation:

Integrating mindfulness and intentional breathing into isometric training fosters a relaxed state of mind, reducing overall stress levels.

4. Positive Mood and Mindset:

The combination of mindfulness and isometrics can contribute to a positive mood and mindset, enhancing your overall well-being.

5. Holistic Approach to Fitness:

The mind-body connection in isometric training aligns with a holistic approach to fitness, addressing both physical and mental dimensions.

Chapter 8

Isometrics Anytime, Anywhere

Isometric Exercises at Home

Welcome to a versatile and accessible chapter that brings isometric exercises to the comfort of your home. In this segment of our isometric journey, we'll explore a range of exercises that require minimal space and no specialized equipment. Whether you're a busy professional, a stay-at-home parent, or simply prefer the convenience of home workouts, this chapter provides you with a toolkit of isometric exercises that can be performed anytime, anywhere.

Isometric Exercises at Home

The beauty of isometric exercises lies in their adaptability and simplicity. You don't need a gym membership or fancy equipment to engage in effective isometric training. The following isometric exercises are designed to target various muscle groups and can be seamlessly incorporated into your home workout routine:

1. Wall Sit:

How to:

Stand with your back against a wall and lower your body into a seated position, forming a 90-degree angle with your knees. Hold the position for the desired duration.

2. *Plank:*

How to:

Assume a push-up position, arms straight beneath your shoulders, and maintain a straight line from head to heels. Hold the plank position for the desired duration.

3. *Static Lunge Hold:*

How to:

Take a step forward with one foot, lowering your body into a lunge position. Hold the static lunge with your front knee forming a 90-degree angle. Switch legs and repeat.

4. *Door Frame Row Hold:*

How to:

Stand facing a door frame, grasp the sides at shoulder height, and lean back, maintaining a straight body. Hold the position, engaging your upper back muscles.

5. *Desk Push-Up Hold:*

How to:

Place your hands on the edge of a sturdy desk, arms shoulder-width apart. Lower your chest toward the desk, pause, and hold the midpoint position.

6. *Seated Leg Press Against Wall:*

How to:

Sit against a wall with your knees bent at a 90-degree angle. Extend one leg, pressing it against the wall, and hold for the desired duration. Switch legs and repeat.

7. *Chair Squat Hold:*

How to:

Stand in front of a chair with feet hip-width apart. Lower your body into a squatting position until you nearly touch the chair. Hold the squat position for the desired duration.

8. *Wrist Contractions:*

How to:

Extend your arms in front of you at shoulder height, palms facing down. Contract your wrist muscles by pressing your fingertips against each other, holding the contraction for the desired duration.

Benefits of Isometrics at Home:

1. Convenience and Time-Efficiency:

Perform isometric exercises at home without the need for additional equipment or travel, making your workouts convenient and time-efficient.

2. Adaptability to Busy Schedules:

Fit in isometric exercises during short breaks or moments of downtime, allowing you to adapt your workout to even the busiest schedules.

3. Minimal Space Requirements:

Isometric exercises at home require minimal space, making them suitable for individuals with limited workout areas.

4. Accessible to All Fitness Levels:

   Whether you're a beginner or an advanced fitness enthusiast, isometrics at home can be tailored to your fitness level, providing a scalable and accessible workout.

5. Consistent Progress Tracking:

  Track your progress easily by monitoring the duration of your isometric holds, allowing you to set goals and consistently challenge yourself.

Sample Home Isometric Routine:

Perform each exercise for 3 sets with a 30-second hold for beginners, progressing to 60 seconds or more for advanced practitioners.

1. Wall Sit - 3 sets of 30 seconds
2. Plank - 3 sets of 30 seconds
3. Static Lunge Hold (each leg) - 3 sets of 30 seconds
4. Door Frame Row Hold - 3 sets of 30 seconds
5. Desk Push-Up Hold - 3 sets of 30 seconds
6. Seated Leg Press Against Wall (each leg) - 3 sets of 30 seconds
7. Chair Squat Hold - 3 sets of 30 seconds
8. Wrist Contractions - 3 sets of 30 seconds

Safety Considerations:
- Ensure the stability of surfaces and furniture used for isometric exercises.
- Focus on maintaining proper form to prevent injuries, especially when performing exercises near furniture or walls.

As we continue our isometric journey, subsequent chapters will explore advanced techniques and specialized routines, ensuring a well-rounded and progressively challenging fitness experience. Onward to achieving your fitness goals right from the comfort of your home!

Isometrics in the Office or Workplace

Welcome to a chapter designed to bring the benefits of isometrics into your workplace. In this segment of our isometric journey, we'll explore quick and discreet routines that can be seamlessly incorporated into your office environment. Whether you're dealing with a hectic work schedule or spend long hours at a desk, these isometric exercises will help you stay active and energized throughout the workday.

Isometrics in the Office or Workplace

Transform your workplace into a fitness-friendly environment by integrating isometric exercises.* The following routines are tailored to accommodate the constraints of an office setting, offering effective workouts that can be completed in a short amount of time. Feel free to incorporate these exercises into your daily routine to boost energy levels, improve focus, and enhance overall well-being.

1. Desk Plank:

How to:

Place your hands on the edge of your desk, arms extended, and walk your feet back until your body forms a straight line. Hold the plank position for 30 seconds to 1 minute.

2. *Chair Squats:*

How to:

Stand in front of your chair, feet hip-width apart. Lower your body into a squatting position, almost touching the chair. Hold the squat for 30 seconds.

3. *Desk Push-Up:*

How to:

Place your hands on the edge of your desk, arms shoulder-width apart. Lower your chest towards the desk, hold the midpoint position for 30 seconds.

4. *Seated Leg Press:*

How to:

Sit comfortably in your chair with feet flat on the floor. Extend one leg, pressing it against the floor, and hold for 30 seconds. Switch legs and repeat.

5. *Wrist Contractions:*

How to:

Extend your arms in front of you at shoulder height, palms facing down. Contract your wrist muscles by pressing your fingertips against each other, holding for 30 seconds.

6. *Wall Sit:*

How to:

Find a clear wall space. Lower your body into a seated position against the wall, forming a 90-degree angle with your knees. Hold the wall sit for 30 seconds to 1 minute.

Quick Isometric Routines for Busy Schedules

These quick routines are designed to seamlessly fit into your workday, allowing you to stay active and maintain energy levels.

Routine 1: Desk Energizer

1. Desk Plank - 1 minute
2. Wrist Contractions - 30 seconds
3. Seated Leg Press - 1 minute (30 seconds per leg)
4. Repeat the circuit twice for a quick, effective workout.

Routine 2: Office Power Break

1. Chair Squats - 1 minute
2. Wall Sit - 1 minute
3. Desk Push-Up - 30 seconds
4. Repeat the circuit twice to re-energize during a break.

Benefits of Isometrics in the Workplace:

1. Boosted Energy Levels:
   Incorporating isometrics at the office helps combat fatigue and boosts energy levels, enhancing productivity and focus.

2. Improved Posture:

Isometric exercises, especially those targeting the core and back muscles, contribute to improved posture, reducing the risk of stiffness.

3. Quick Stress Relief:

A short isometric routine provides a quick break from work stress, promoting mental clarity and relaxation.

4. Increased Circulation:

Engaging in isometrics stimulates blood flow, preventing the negative effects of prolonged sitting and promoting overall circulation.

5. Discreet and Time-Efficient:

Isometrics can be performed discreetly, making them suitable for the office, and they require minimal time, making them feasible even in busy schedules.

Safety Considerations:
- Be mindful of your surroundings and ensure your workspace is clear before starting isometric exercises.
- Adjust the duration of holds based on your fitness level and comfort.

As we progress in our isometric journey, subsequent chapters will explore advanced techniques and integrative routines to continue enhancing your fitness experience. Onward to incorporating isometrics seamlessly into your workday for a healthier and more energized you!

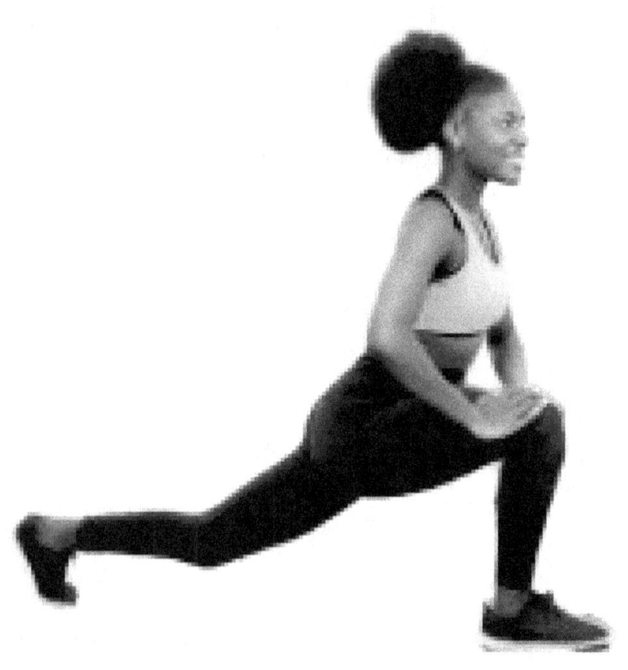

Conclusion

As we draw the final pages of our journey together, it's a moment of reflection and celebration. Throughout this book, "Isometric Exercises for Pain Relief: Relieve Aches in Your Back, Neck, Knees and More Using Simple Static Contraction Exercises Without Equipment," we've explored the transformative power of isometrics in not only alleviating pain but also in unlocking strength and vitality.

In the beginning, we embarked on a mission to discover the untapped potential within our muscles, the potential to mend and fortify. Isometric exercises became our allies, guiding us through static holds that not only targeted pain points but also sculpted a resilient foundation for overall well-being.

From the foundational chapters that introduced us to the basics, to the advanced techniques that challenged our limits, we have witnessed the evolution of our fitness journey. We learned that isometrics isn't just a set of exercises; it's a philosophy, a mindful approach to movement that connects the body and mind in harmony.

The chapters on targeting specific aches and pains became maps, guiding us to relief. From back pain to knee discomfort, each section was a compass directing us toward a pain-free existence. And as we navigated, we discovered the joy of customization, tailoring isometric exercises to our fitness levels, making them an integral part of our daily routines.

The workplace and home transformed into our fitness arenas, where quick, efficient isometric routines became our secret weapons against the sedentary effects of modern life. We harnessed the power of isometrics in the office, turning moments of stillness into opportunities for strength-building and stress relief.

But beyond the physical, we delved into the mind-body connection, where mindfulness and intentional breathing merged seamlessly with isometrics, offering a holistic approach to our well-being. Stress found its match in the deliberate holds and controlled breaths, creating a serene sanctuary within the dynamic world of isometrics.

Now, as we conclude this chapter of our journey, let's carry forward the lessons of strength, resilience, and mindfulness. Let the isometric revolution be a continuous narrative in our lives, a testament to the incredible potential within each one of us. The echoes of our static holds will resonate in the days to come, reminding us that strength is not just a physical attribute but a state of being.

May the pain relief experienced through these pages be the catalyst for a life filled with movement, vigor, and the joy of an empowered existence. As you close this book, remember, the journey doesn't end here; it's a continuum of discovery, growth, and the unwavering pursuit of a pain-free, powerful life.

www.ingramcontent.com/pod-product-compliance
Lightning Source LLC
Chambersburg PA
CBHW071055260726
48661CB00006B/2289